# The Complete

# Fryer Cookbook for good

# dessert

*50 low-carb air fryer delicious dessert recipes, easy to prepare to lose weight and burn fat fast*

*Kate Mitchell*

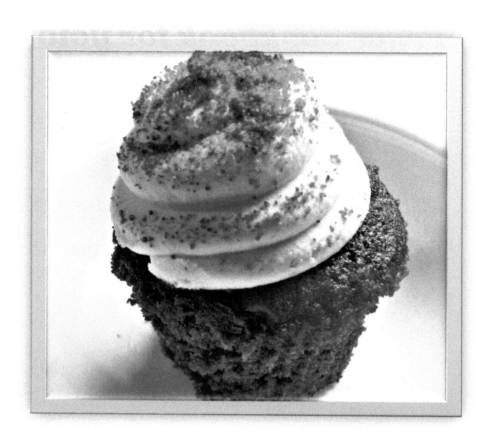

3

sources. Please consult a licensed professional before attempting any techniques outlined in this book.

By reading this document, the reader agrees that under no circumstances is the author responsible for any losses, direct or indirect, which are incurred as a result of the use of information contained within this document, including, but not limited to, — errors, omissions, or inaccuracies.

# Table of contents

# INTRODUCTION

Out there, many diets aim to help you lose weight. Some of them work, too! This does not justify, however, the vast number of dieters who struggle to achieve their targets. Oh, why is that? Is dieting that hard? Or is something else going on that causes them to neglect their objectives?

The truth is that dieting is difficult. When you try to get better and lose weight, you try to reverse years of patterns that won't vanish unexpectedly. For this reason, many dieters report gaining the weight they lost right back once. The dieting experience stresses them to such a degree that they start binge eating and undo all the good work they have done until they stop dieting. No one right way to diet exists. The trick to dieting is to follow a successful strategy and then make it as simple as possible to follow what needs to be achieved. The thing to keep in mind is that not all diets can be adopted easily. This is not due to any ambiguity within them. It's just that certain individuals are used to eating in the way prescribed by the diet. One such example is the ketogenic diet. The diet calls for the intake of a very limited amount of carbohydrates. This means food is off the menu, such as rice, pasta, and other starchy vegetables such as potatoes. Also, relaxed variations of the keto diet dramatically reduce carbohydrates, undermining the aims of several dieters.

To adopt the diet, they end up having to exert massive quantities of willpower.

As willpower is like a muscle, this doesn't do them any favors. It tires at some stage, and this is when the dieter goes right back to their old eating routine. With that, I have personal knowledge. The keto diet provides the most in terms of health benefits. Carbohydrate reduction forces the body to mobilize fat, resulting in automatic fat loss and improved health.

Although the benefits were huge, I could not adhere to the diet for long periods because of lifestyle problems. The truth is that I was incredibly busy and didn't have time to spend in the kitchen when I started on the keto diet. Not only did I lack time, I had no desire to be there. As far as I was concerned, one that could make a great dish in a few minutes was the best recipe! You probably know how much of the recipe works if you have adopted the keto diet. Grilling and baking are involved in most of them. Then they put the protein in a salad, and that's your dinner. Although the novelty factor succeeded in keeping me excited about meals, it soon wore off.

Before they become disgusting, there's only so much salad a person can consume! No amount of fancy meat and vegetables will make them more appealing. I need a stronger solution.

One of a million people's favorite diets is the Keto diet. How to make your food simpler and pleasant are different secrets and lifehacks. Everyone knows that only tasty food will offer us a healthy mood and pleasure. But, it can be a little hard to maintain the following diet. However, nothing is impossible. With the name "Keto Air Fryer Cooking," this book will open up the secret to you. Just imagine that you will eat crunchy, tasty, and tender food without a huge amount of oil in it. Will a fairy tale look like that? It comes real with this book and air fryer. If we fry it, there are a lot of meals that will be more delicious. But we used to know that they can steam or boil nutritious food. Air fryer is a magic appliance that can cook your favorite meals with the minimum amount of fat simply and safely.

This kitchen tool has hundreds of advantages: it is easy to use and can be used as adults, elderly people, or even teenagers do; it can replace other kitchen appliances; the cooking time is less compared to ordinary time. The benefits of an air fryer can be mentioned, but starting to cook is better! This book will teach you how to cook fabulous meals healthily and simply! Let's get started!

# Angel Food Cake

**Prep Time** 10 m | **Cook Time** 30 m | 12 **Servings**

- ¼ cup butter, melted

- 1 cup powdered erythritol

- 1 teaspoon strawberry extract

- 12 egg whites

- 2 teaspoons cream of tartar

- A pinch of salt

1. Preheat the air fryer for 5 minutes.

2. Mix the egg whites with the cream of tartar.

3. Use a hand mixer and whisk until white and fluffy.

4. Add the rest of the ingredients except for the butter and whisk for another minute.

5. Pour into a baking dish.

6. Place in the oven basket and cook for 30 minutes at 4000F, or if a toothpick inserted in the middle comes out clean.

7. Drizzle with melted butter once cooled.

**Per Serving:** Calories 65|Carbohydrates 1.8g|Protein 3.1g|Fat 5g

# Apple Pie in Air Fryer

**Prep Time** 15 m | Cooking Time 35 m | 4 Servings

- ½ teaspoon vanilla extract

- 1 beaten egg

- 1 large apple, chopped

- 1 Pillsbury Refrigerator pie crust

- 1 tablespoon butter

- 1 tablespoon ground cinnamon

- 1 tablespoon raw sugar

- 2 tablespoon sugar

- 2 teaspoons lemon juice

- Baking spray

1. Lightly grease the baking pan of the air fryer with cooking spray. Spread the pie crust on the rare part of the pan up to the sides.

2. In a bowl, make a mixture of vanilla, sugar, cinnamon, lemon juice, and apples. Pour on top of pie crust. Top apples with butter slices.

3. Cover apples with the other pie crust. Pierce with a knife the tops of the pie.

4. Spread whisked egg on top of crust and sprinkle sugar.

5. Cover with foil.

6. For 25 minutes, cook at 390oF.

7. Remove foil cook for 10 minutes at 330oF until tops are browned.

**Per Serving:** Calories 372|Carbs 44.7g|Protein 4.2g|Fat 19.6g

# Apple-Toffee Upside-Down Cake

**Prep Time** 10 m | P Cooking Time 30 m | 9 Servings

- ¼ cup almond butter

- ¼ cup sunflower oil

- ½ cup walnuts, chopped

- ¾ cup + 3 tablespoon coconut sugar

- ¾ cup water

- 1 ½ teaspoon mixed spice

- 1 cup plain flour

- 1 lemon, zest

- 1 teaspoon baking soda

- 1 teaspoon vinegar

- 3 baking apples, cored and sliced

1. Preheat the air fryer to 390oF.

2. In a skillet, melt the almond butter and 3 tablespoons of sugar. Pour the mixture over a baking dish that will fit in the air fryer. Arrange the slices of apples on top. Set aside.

3. In a mixing bowl, combine flour, ¾ cup sugar, and baking soda. Add the mixed spice.

4. In a different bowl, mix the water, oil, vinegar, and lemon zest. Stir in the chopped walnuts.

5. Combine the wet ingredients to the dry ingredients until well combined.

6. Pour over the tin with apple slices.

7. Bake for 30 minutes or until a toothpick inserted comes out clean.

**Per Serving:** Calories 335 |Carbohydrates 39.6g | Protein 3.8g | Fat 17.9g

# Banana-Choco Brownies

**Prep Time** 15 m | **Cook Time** 30 m | 12 **Servings**

- 2 cups almond flour
- 2 teaspoons baking powder
- ½ teaspoon baking powder
- ½ teaspoon baking soda
- ½ teaspoon salt
- 1 over-ripe banana
- 3 large eggs
- ½ teaspoon stevia powder
- ¼ cup coconut oil
- 1 tablespoon vinegar
- 1/3 cup almond flour
- 1/3 cup cocoa powder

1. Preheat the air fryer for 5 minutes.

2. Add together all ingredients in a food processor and pulse until well combined.

3. Pour into a skillet that will fit in the deep fryer.

4. Place in the fryer basket and cook for 30 minutes at 3500F, or if a toothpick inserted in the middle comes out clean.

**Per Serving:** Calories 75|Carbohydrates 2.1g |Protein 1.7g|Fat 6.6g

# Blueberry & Lemon Cake

**Prep Time** 10 m | **Cook Time** 17 m | 4 **Servings**

- 2 eggs

- 1 cup blueberries

- zest from 1 lemon

- juice from 1 lemon

- 1 tsp. vanilla

- brown sugar for topping (a little sprinkling on top of each muffin-less than a teaspoon)

- 2 1/2 cups self-rising flour

- 1/2 cup Monk Fruit (or use your preferred sugar)

- 1/2 cup cream

- 1/4 cup avocado oil (any light cooking oil)

1. In a mixing bowl, beat well the wet ingredients. Stir in dry ingredients and mix thoroughly.

2. Lightly grease the baking pan of the air fryer with cooking spray. Pour in batter.

3. For 12 minutes, cook at 330F.

4. Let it stand in the air fryer for 5 minutes.

**Per Serving:** Calories 589|Carbs 76.7g|Protein 13.5g|Fat 25.3g

# Bread Pudding with Cranberry

**Prep Time** 20 m | Cooking Time 45 m | 4 Servings

- 1-1/2 cups milk

- 2-1/2 eggs

- 1/2 cup cranberries1 teaspoon butter

- 1/4 cup golden raisins

- 1/8 teaspoon ground cinnamon

- 3/4 cup heavy whipping cream

- 3/4 teaspoon lemon zest

- 3/4 teaspoon kosher salt

- 2 tbsp. and 1/4 cup white sugar

- 3/4 French baguettes, cut into 2-inch slices 3/8 vanilla bean, split and seeds scraped away

1. Lightly grease the baking pan of the air fryer with cooking spray. Spread baguette slices, cranberries, and raisins.

2. In a blender, blend well vanilla bean, cinnamon, salt, lemon zest, eggs, sugar, and cream. Pour over baguette slices. Let it soak for an hour.

3. Cover pan with foil.

4. For 35 minutes, cook at 330F.

5. Let it rest for 10 minutes.


**Per Serving:** Calories 581 |Carbs 76.1g|Protein 15.8g|Fat 23.7g

# Cherries 'n Almond Flour Bars

**Prep Time** 15 m | **Cook Time** 35 m | 12 **Servings**

- ¼ cup of water

- ½ cup butter softened

- ½ teaspoon salt

- ½ teaspoon vanilla

- 1 ½ cups almond flour

- 1 cup erythritol

- 1 cup fresh cherries, pitted

- 1 tablespoon xanthan gum

- 2 eggs

1. In a medium bowl, make a mixture of the first 6 ingredients to form a dough.

2. Press the batter onto a baking sheet that will fit in the air fryer.

3. Place in the fryer and bake for 10 minutes at 375F.

4. Meanwhile, mix the cherries, water, and xanthan gum in a bowl.

5. Scoop out the dough and pour over the cherry.

6. Return to the fryer and cook for another 25 minutes at 3750F.

**Per Serving:** Calories 99 |Carbohydrates 2.1g |Protein 1.8g|Fat 9.3g

# Cherry-Choco Bars

**Prep Time** 5 m | **Cook Time** 15 m | 8 **Servings**

- ¼ teaspoon salt

- ½ cup almonds, sliced

- ½ cup chia seeds

- ½ cup dark chocolate, chopped

- ½ cup dried cherries, chopped

- ½ cup prunes, pureed

- ½ cup quinoa, cooked

- ¾ cup almond butter

- 1/3 cup honey

- 2 cups old-fashioned oats

- 2 tablespoon coconut oil

1. Preheat the air fryer to 375OF.

2. In a bowl, combine the oats, quinoa, chia seeds, almond, cherries, and chocolate.

3. In a saucepan, heat the almond butter, honey, and coconut oil.

4. Pour the butter mixture over the dry mixture. Add salt and prunes.

5. Mix until well combined.

6. Pour over a baking dish that can fit inside the air fryer.

7. Cook for 15 minutes.

8. Allow settling for an hour before slicing into bars.

**Per Serving:** Calories 321|Carbohydrates 35g|Protein 7g|Fat 17g

# Chocolate Chip in a Mug

**Prep Time** 10 m | **Cook Time** 20 m | 6 **Servings**

- ¼ cup walnuts, shelled and chopped

- ½ cup butter, unsalted

- ½ cup dark chocolate chips

- ½ cup erythritol

- ½ teaspoon baking soda

- ½ teaspoon salt

- 1 tablespoon vanilla extract

- 2 ½ cups almond flour

- 2 large eggs, beaten

1. Preheat the air fryer for 5 minutes.

2. Combine all ingredients in a mixing bowl.

3. Place in greased mugs.

4. Bake in the air fryer oven for 20 minutes at 375OF.

**Per Serving:** Calories 234|Carbohydrates 4.9g|Protein 2.3g|Fat 22.8g

# Choco-Peanut Mug Cake

**Prep Time** 10 m | **Cook Time** 20 m | 6 **Servings**

- ¼ teaspoon baking powder

- ½ teaspoon vanilla extract

- 1 egg

- 1 tablespoon heavy cream

- 1 tablespoon peanut butter

- 1 teaspoon butter, softened

- 2 tablespoon erythritol

- 2 tablespoons cocoa powder, unsweetened

1. Preheat the air fryer for 5 minutes.

2. Combine all ingredients in a mixing bowl.

3. Pour into a greased mug.

4. Place in the air fryer oven basket and cook for 20 minutes at 4000F, or if a toothpick inserted in the middle comes out clean.

**Per Serving:** Calories 293 |Carbohydrates 8.5g|Protein 12.4g|Fat 23.3g

# Coco-Lime Bars

**Prep Time** 10 m | **Cook Time** 20 m | 3 **Servings**

- ¼ cup almond flour

- ¼ cup coconut oil

- ¼ cup dried coconut flakes

- ¼ teaspoon salt

- ½ cup lime juice

- ¾ cup coconut flour

- 1 ¼ cup erythritol powder

- 1 tablespoon lime zest

- 4 eggs

1. Preheat the air fryer for 5 minutes.

2. Combine all ingredients in a mixing bowl.

3. Place in the greased mug.

4. Bake in the air fryer oven for 20 minutes at 375F.

**Per Serving:** Calories 506 | Carbohydrates 21.9g| Protein 19.3g | Fat 37.9g

# Coconut 'n Almond Fat Bombs

**Prep Time** 5 m | Cooking Time 15 m | 12 Servings

- ¼ cup almond flour
- ½ cup shredded coconut
- 1 tablespoon coconut oil
- 1 tablespoon vanilla extract
- 2 tablespoons liquid stevia
- 3 egg whites

1. Preheat the air fryer for 5 minutes.

2. Combine all ingredients in a mixing bowl.

3. Form small balls using your hands.

4. Place in the air fryer oven basket and cook for 15 minutes at 400oF.

**Per Serving:** Calories 23 |Carbohydrates 0.7g|Protein 1.1g|Fat 1.8g

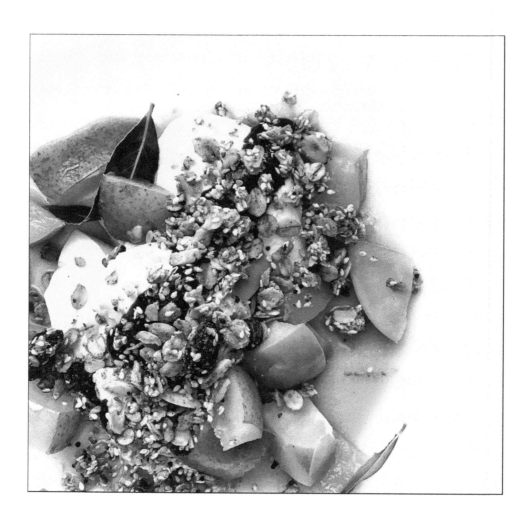

# Coconutty Lemon Bars

**Prep Time** 10 m | **Cook Time** 25 m | 12 **Servings**

- ¼ cup cashew

- ¼ cup fresh lemon juice, freshly squeezed

- ¾ cup coconut milk

- ¾ cup erythritol

- 1 cup desiccated coconut

- 1 teaspoon baking powder

- 2 eggs, beaten

- 2 tablespoons coconut oil

- A dash of salt

1. Preheat the air fryer for 5 minutes.

2. In a mixing bowl, combine all ingredients.

3. Use a hand mixer to mix everything.

4. Pour into a baking bowl that will fit in the air fryer.

5. Bake for 25 minutes at 350F or until a toothpick inserted in the middle comes out clean.

**Per Serving:** Calories 118|Carbohydrates 3.9g|Protein 2.6g |Fat 10.2g

# Coffee 'n Blueberry Cake

**Prep Time** 15 m | **Cook Time** 35 m | 6 **Servings**

- 1 cup white sugar

- 1 egg

- 1/2 cup butter, softened

- 1/2 cup fresh or frozen blueberries

- 1/2 cup sour cream

- 1/2 teaspoon baking powder

- 1/2 teaspoon ground cinnamon

- 1/2 teaspoon vanilla extract

- 1/4 cup brown sugar

- 1/4 cup chopped pecans

- 1/8 teaspoon salt

- 1-1/2 teaspoons confectioners' sugar for dusting

- 3/4 cup and 1 tablespoon all-purpose flour

1. In a small bowl, whisk well pecans, cinnamon, and brown sugar.

2. In a blender, blend well all wet ingredients. Add dry ingredients except for confectioner's sugar and blueberries. Blend well until smooth and creamy.

3. Lightly grease the baking pan of the air fryer with cooking spray.

4. Pour half of the batter into the pan. Sprinkle a little of the pecan mixture on top. Pour the remaining batter and then top with the remaining pecan mixture.

5. Cover pan with foil.

6. For 35 minutes, cook at 330oF.

7. Serve and enjoy with a dusting of confectioner's sugar.


**Per Serving:** Calories 471|Carbs 59.5g|Protein 4.1g |Fat 24.0g

# Coffee Flavored Cookie Dough

**Prep Time** 10 m | **Cook Time** 20 m | 12 **Servings**

- ¼ cup butter

- ¼ teaspoon xanthan gum

- ½ teaspoon coffee espresso powder

- ½ teaspoon stevia powder

- ¾ cup almond flour

- 1 egg

- 1 teaspoon vanilla

- 1/3 cup sesame seeds

- 2 tablespoons cocoa powder

- 2 tablespoons cream cheese, softened

1. Preheat the air fryer for 5 minutes.

2. Combine all ingredients in a mixing bowl.

3. Press into a baking dish that will fit in the air fryer.

4. Place in the air fryer oven basket and cook for 20 minutes at 4000F, or if a toothpick inserted in the middle comes out clean.

**Per Serving:** Calories 88|Carbohydrates 1.3g|Protein 1.9g|Fat 8.3g

# Angel Food Cake

**Prep Time** 10 m | **Cook Time** 30 m | 12 **Servings**

- ¼ cup butter, melted

- 1 cup powdered erythritol

- 1 teaspoon strawberry extract

- egg whites

- teaspoons cream of tartar

- A pinch of salt

1. Preheat the air fryer for 5 minutes.

2. Mix the egg whites with the cream of tartar.

3. Use a hand mixer and whisk until white and fluffy.

4. Add the rest of the ingredients except for the butter and whisk for another minute.

5. Pour into a baking dish.

6. Place in the oven basket and cook for 30 minutes at 4000F, or if a toothpick inserted in the middle comes out clean.

7. Drizzle with melted butter once cooled.

**Per Serving:** Calories: 65 |Carbohydrates: 1.8g |Protein: 3.1g |Fat: 5g

# Apple Pie in Air Fryer

**Prep Time** 15 m | **Cook Time** 35 m | 4 **Servings**

- ½ teaspoon vanilla extract
- 1 beaten egg
- 1 large apple, chopped
- 1 Pillsbury Refrigerator pie crust
- 1 tablespoon butter
- 1 tablespoon ground cinnamon
- 1 tablespoon raw sugar
- tablespoon sugar
- teaspoons lemon juice
- Baking spray

1.Lightly grease the baking pan of the air fryer with cooking spray. Spread pie crust on rare part of the pan up to the sides.

2.In a bowl, make a mixture of vanilla, sugar, cinnamon, lemon juice, and apples. Pour on top of pie crust. Top apples with butter slices.

3.Cover apples with the other pie crust. Pierce with a knife the tops of the pie.

4.Spread whisked egg on top of crust and sprinkle sugar.

5.Cover with foil.

6.For 25 minutes, cook on 3900F.

7.Remove foil cook for 10 minutes at 3300F until tops are browned.


**Per Serving:** Calories 372 |Carbs: 44.7g |Protein: 4.2g| Fat: 19.6g

# Apple-Toffee Upside-Down Cake

**Prep Time** 10 m | **Cook Time** 30 m | 9 **Servings**

- ¼ cup almond butter

- ¼ cup sunflower oil

- ½ cup walnuts, chopped

- ¾ cup + 3 tablespoon coconut sugar

- ¾ cup water

- 1 ½ teaspoon mixed spice

- 1 cup plain flour

- 1 lemon, zest

- 1 teaspoon baking soda

- 1 teaspoon vinegar

- baking apples, cored and sliced

1.Preheat the air fryer to 390oF.

2. In a skillet, melt the almond butter and 3 tablespoons of sugar. Pour the mixture over a baking dish that will fit in the air fryer. Arrange the slices of apples on top. Set aside.

3. In a mixing bowl, combine flour, ¾ cup sugar, and baking soda. Add the mixed spice.

4. In a different bowl, mix the water, oil, vinegar, and lemon zest. Stir in the chopped walnuts.

5. Combine the wet ingredients to the dry ingredients until well combined.

6. Pour over the tin with apple slices.

7. Bake for 30 minutes or until a toothpick inserted comes out clean.

**Per Serving:** Calories: 335| Carbohydrates: 39.6g |Protein: 3.8g| Fat: 17.9g

# Banana-Choco Brownies

**Prep Time** 15 m | **Cook Time** 30 m | 12 **Servings**

- cups almond flour
- teaspoons baking powder
- ½ teaspoon baking powder
- ½ teaspoon baking soda
- ½ teaspoon salt
- 1 over-ripe banana
- large eggs
- ½ teaspoon stevia powder
- ¼ cup coconut oil
- 1 tablespoon vinegar
- 1/3 cup almond flour
- 1/3 cup cocoa powder

1. Preheat the air fryer for 5 minutes.

2. Add together all ingredients in a food processor and pulse until well combined.

3. Pour into a skillet that will fit in the deep fryer.

4. Place in the fryer basket and cook for 30 minutes at 3500F, or if a toothpick inserted in the middle comes out clean.

**Per Serving:** Calories: 75 |Carbohydrates: 2.1g| Protein: 1.7g |Fat: 6.6g

# Blueberry & Lemon Cake

**Prep Time** 10 m | **Cook Time** 17 m | 4 **Servings**

- eggs

- 1 cup blueberries

- Zest from 1 lemon

- Juice from 1 lemon

- 1 tsp. vanilla

- Brown sugar for topping (a little sprinkling on top of each muffin-less than a teaspoon)

- 1/2 cups self-rising flour

- 1/2 cup Monk Fruit (or use your preferred sugar)

- 1/2 cup cream

- 1/4 cup avocado oil (any light cooking oil)

1.In a mixing bowl, beat well-wet Ingredients. Stir in dry ingredients and mix thoroughly.

49

2.Lightly grease the baking pan of the air fryer with cooking spray. Pour in batter.

3.For 12 minutes, cook on 3300F.

4.Let it stand in the air fryer for 5 minutes.


**Per Serving:** Calories: 589| Carbs: 76.7g |Protein: 13.5g |Fat: 25.3g

# Chocolate Chip in a Mug

**Prep Time** 10 m | **Cook Time** 20 m | 6 **Servings**

- ¼ cup walnuts, shelled and chopped

- ½ cup butter, unsalted

- ½ cup dark chocolate chips

- ½ cup erythritol

- ½ teaspoon baking soda

- ½ teaspoon salt

- 1 tablespoon vanilla extract

- ½ cups almond flour

- large eggs, beaten

1.Preheat the air fryer for 5 minutes.

2.Combine all ingredients in a mixing bowl.

3.Place in greased mugs.

4.Bake in the air fryer oven for 20 minutes at 375oF.

**Per Serving:** Calories: 234| Carbohydrates: 4.9g |Protein:

2.3g |Fat: 22.8g

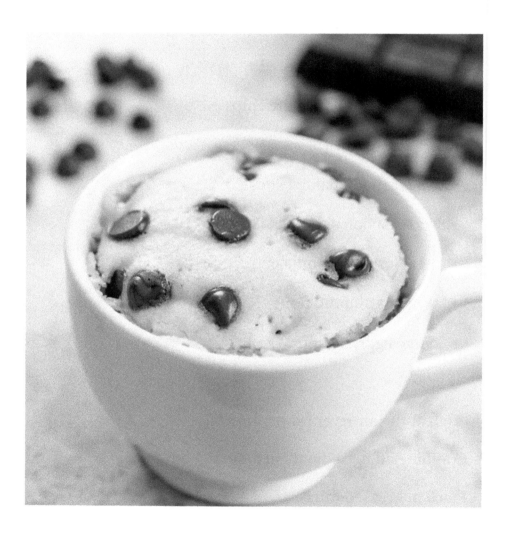

# Bread Pudding with Cranberry

**Prep Time** 20 m | **Cook Time** 45 m | 4 **Servings**

- 1-1/2 cups milk

- 2-1/2 eggs

- 1/2 cup cranberries1 teaspoon butter

- 1/4 cup golden raisins

- 1/8 teaspoon ground cinnamon

- 3/4 cup heavy whipping cream

- 3/4 teaspoon lemon zest

- 3/4 teaspoon kosher salt

- tbsp. and 1/4 cup white sugar

- 3/4 French baguettes, cut into 2-inch slices 3/8 vanilla bean, split and seeds scraped away

1.Lightly grease the baking pan of the air fryer with cooking spray. Spread baguette slices, cranberries, and raisins.

2.In a blender, blend well vanilla bean, cinnamon, salt, lemon zest, eggs, sugar, and cream. Pour over baguette slices. Let it soak for an hour.

3.Cover pan with foil.

4.For 35 minutes, cook on 330oF.

5.Let it rest for 10 minutes.

**Per Serving:** Calories: 581 |Carbs: 76.1g |Protein: 15.8g |Fat: 23.7g

# Cherries 'n Almond Flour Bars

**Prep Time** 15 m | **Cook Time** 35 m | 12 **Servings**

- ¼ cup of water
- ½ cup butter softened
- ½ teaspoon salt
- ½ teaspoon vanilla
- 1 ½ cups almond flour
- 1 cup erythritol
- 1 cup fresh cherries, pitted
- 1 tablespoon xanthan gum
- eggs

1.In a medium bowl, make a mixture of the first 6 ingredients to form a dough.

2.Press the batter onto a baking sheet that will fit in the air fryer.

3.Place in the fryer and bake for 10 minutes at 375OF.

4.Meanwhile, mix the cherries, water, and xanthan gum in a bowl.

5. Scoop out the dough and pour over the cherry.

6.Return to the fryer and cook for another 25 minutes at 375OF.


**Per Serving:** Calories: 99 |Carbohydrates: 2.1g |Protein: 1.8g |Fat: 9.3g

# Cherry-Choco Bars

**Prep Time** 5 m | **Cook Time** 15 m | 8 **Servings**

- ¼ teaspoon salt

- ½ cup almonds, sliced

- ½ cup chia seeds

- ½ cup dark chocolate, chopped

- ½ cup dried cherries, chopped

- ½ cup prunes, pureed

- ½ cup quinoa, cooked

- ¾ cup almond butter

- 1/3 cup honey

- cups old-fashioned oats

- tablespoon coconut oil

1.Preheat the air fryer to 375oF.

2.In a bowl, combine the oats, quinoa, chia seeds, almond, cherries, and chocolate.

3.In a saucepan, heat the almond butter, honey, and coconut oil.

4.Pour the butter mixture over the dry mixture. Add salt and prunes.

5.Mix until well combined.

6.Pour over a baking dish that can fit inside the air fryer.

7.Cook for 15 minutes.

8.Allow settling for an hour before slicing into bars.

**Per Serving:** Calories: 321 |Carbohydrates: 35g |Protein: 7g |Fat: 17g

# Choco-Peanut Mug Cake

**Prep Time** 10 m | **Cook Time** 20 m | 6 **Servings**

- ¼ teaspoon baking powder

- ½ teaspoon vanilla extract

- 1 egg

- 1 tablespoon heavy cream

- 1 tablespoon peanut butter

- 1 teaspoon butter, softened

- tablespoon erythritol

- tablespoons cocoa powder, unsweetened

1.Preheat the air fryer for 5 minutes.

2.Combine all ingredients in a mixing bowl.

3.Pour into a greased mug.

4.Place in the air fryer oven basket and cook for 20 minutes at 4000F, or if a toothpick inserted in the middle comes out clean.

**Per Serving:** Calories: 293 |Carbohydrates: 8.5g |Protein: 12.4g |Fat: 23.3g

# Coco-Lime Bars

**Prep Time** 10 m | **Cook Time** 20 m | 3 **Servings**

- ¼ cup almond flour

- ¼ cup coconut oil

- ¼ cup dried coconut flakes

- ¼ teaspoon salt

- ½ cup lime juice

- ¾ cup coconut flour

- 1 ¼ cup erythritol powder

- 1 tablespoon lime zest

- eggs

1. Preheat the air fryer for 5 minutes.

2. Combine all ingredients in a mixing bowl.

3. Place in the greased mug.

4. Bake in the air fryer oven for 20 minutes at 375oF.

**Per Serving:** Calories: 506 |Carbohydrates: 21.9g|

Protein: 19.3g |Fat: 37.9g

# Coconut 'n Almond Fat Bombs

**Prep Time** 5 m | **Cook Time** 15 m | 12 **Servings**

- ¼ cup almond flour

- ½ cup shredded coconut

- 1 tablespoon coconut oil

- 1 tablespoon vanilla extract

- tablespoons liquid stevia

- egg whites

1.Preheat the air fryer for 5 minutes.

2.Combine all ingredients in a mixing bowl.

3.Form small balls using your hands.

4.Place in the air fryer oven basket and cook for 15 minutes

at 4000F.

**Per Serving:** Calories: 23 |Carbohydrates: 0.7g |Protein: 1.1g |Fat: 1.8g

# Coconutty Lemon Bars

**Prep Time** 10 m | **Cook Time** 25 m | 12 **Servings**

- ¼ cup cashew

- ¼ cup fresh lemon juice, freshly squeezed

- ¾ cup coconut milk

- ¾ cup erythritol

- 1 cup desiccated coconut

- 1 teaspoon baking powder

- eggs, beaten

- tablespoons coconut oil

- A dash of salt

1. Preheat the air fryer for 5 minutes.

2. In a mixing bowl, combine all ingredients.

3. Use a hand mixer to mix everything.

4. Pour into a baking bowl that will fit in the air fryer.

5.Bake for 25 minutes at 3500F or until a toothpick inserted in the middle comes out clean.

**Per Serving:** Calories: 118 |Carbohydrates: 3.9g |Protein: 2.6g| Fat: 10.2g

# Coffee 'n Blueberry Cake

**Prep Time** 15 m | **Cook Time** 35 m | 6 **Servings**

- 1 cup white sugar

- 1 egg

- 1/2 cup butter, softened

- 1/2 cup fresh or frozen blueberries

- 1/2 cup sour cream

- 1/2 teaspoon baking powder

- 1/2 teaspoon ground cinnamon

- 1/2 teaspoon vanilla extract

- 1/4 cup brown sugar

- 1/4 cup chopped pecans

- 1/8 teaspoon salt

- 1-1/2 teaspoons confectioners' sugar for dusting

- 3/4 cup and 1 tablespoon all-purpose flour

1. In a small bowl, whisk well pecans, cinnamon, and brown sugar.

2. In a blender, blend well all wet Ingredients. Add dry ingredients except for confectioner's sugar and blueberries. Blend well until smooth and creamy.

3. Lightly grease the baking pan of the air fryer with cooking spray.

4. Pour half of the batter into the pan. Sprinkle small of the pecan mixture on top. Pour the remaining batter. And then topped with the remaining pecan mixture.

5. Cover pan with foil.

6. For 35 minutes, cook on 330oF.

7. Serve and enjoy with a dusting of confectioner's sugar.


**Per Serving:** Calories: 471|Carbs: 59.5g |Protein: 4.1g |Fat: 24.0g

# Coffee Flavored Cookie Dough

**Prep Time** 10 m | **Cook Time** 20 m | 12 **Servings**

- ¼ cup butter

- ¼ teaspoon xanthan gum

- ½ teaspoon coffee espresso powder

- ½ teaspoon stevia powder

- ¾ cup almond flour

- 1 egg

- 1 teaspoon vanilla

- 1/3 cup sesame seeds

- tablespoons cocoa powder

- tablespoons cream cheese softened

1. Preheat the air fryer for 5 minutes.

2. Combine all ingredients in a mixing bowl.

3. Press into a baking dish that will fit in the air fryer.

4. Place in the air fryer oven basket and cook for 20 minutes at 4000F, or if a toothpick inserted in the middle comes out clean.

**Per Serving:** Calories: 88 |Carbohydrates: 1.3g |Protein: 1.9g| Fat: 8.3g

# Sweet Potato Tater Tots

**Prep Time** 10 m | **Cook Time** 23 m | 4 **Servings**

- 1sweet potatoes, peeled
- 1/2 tsp. Cajun seasoning
- Olive oil cooking spray
- Sea salt to taste

1.Boil sweet potatoes in water for 15 minutes over medium-high heat.

2.Drain the sweet potatoes, then allow them to cool

3. Peel the boiled sweet potatoes and return them to the bowl.

4. Mash the potatoes and stir in salt and Cajun seasoning. Mix well and make small tater tots out of it.

5.Place the tater tots in the Air Fryer basket and spray them with cooking oil.

6.Place the Air Fryer basket inside the Air Fryer toaster and close the lid.

7. Select Air Frying mode at a temperature of 400 ° F for 8 minutes.

8. Turn the trays over and continue cooking for another 8 minutes.

**Per Serving:** Calories: 184 Cal |Protein: 9 g |Carbs: 43 g |Fat: 17 g

# Fried Ravioli

**Prep Time** 10 m | **Cook Time** 15 m | 4 **Servings**

- 1 package ravioli, frozen
- 1 cup breadcrumbs
- 1/2 cup parmesan cheese
- 1 tbs. Italian seasoning
- 1 tbs. garlic powder
- Eggs, beaten
- Cooking spray

1. Mix breadcrumbs with garlic powder, cheese, and Italian seasoning in a bowl.

2. Whisk eggs in another bowl. Dip each ravioli in eggs first, then coat them with a crumbs mixture.

3. Place the ravioli in the Air Fryer basket. Place the air Fryer basket inside the oven and close the lid.

4. Select the Air Fry mode at 360°F temperature for 15 minutes.

5. Flip the ravioli after 8 minutes and resume cooking.

**Per Serving:** Calories: 124 Cal |Protein: 4.5 g | Carbs: 27.5 g| Fat: 3.5 g

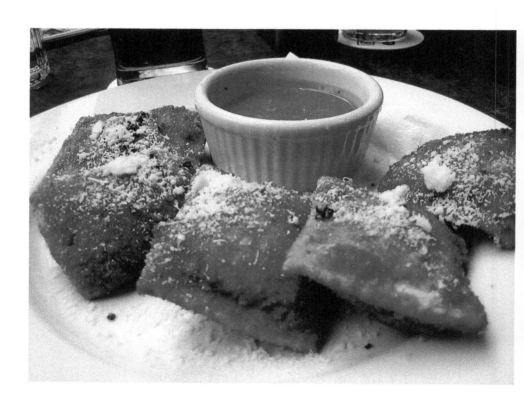

# Eggplant Fries

**Prep Time** 10 m | **Cook Time** 20 m | 4 **Servings**

- 1/2 cup panko breadcrumbs

- 1/2 tsp. salt

- 1 eggplant, peeled and sliced

- 1 cup egg, whisked

1. Toss the breadcrumbs with salt in a tray.

2. Dip the eggplant in the whisked egg and coat with the crumb's mixture.

3.Place the eggplant slices in the Air Fryer basket. Put the basket inside the Air Fryer toaster oven and close the lid.

4.Select the Air Fry mode at 400°F temperature for 20 minutes.

5. Flip the slices after 10 minutes, then resume cooking.

**Per Serving:** Calories: 110 Cal| Protein: 5 g |Carbs: 12.8 g | Fat: 11.9 g

# Stuffed Eggplants

**Prep Time** 10 m | **Cook Time** 38 m | 4 **Servings**

- Eggplants, cut in half lengthwise

- 1/2 cup shredded cheddar cheese

- 1/2 can (7.5 oz.) chili without beans

- 1 Tsp. kosher salt

FOR SERVING

- Tbsp. cooked bacon bits

- tbsp. sour cream

- Fresh scallions, thinly sliced

1. Place the eggplants halves in the Air Fryer toaster oven and close the lid.

2. Select the Air Fry mode at 390°F temperature for 35 minutes.

3. Top each eggplant half with chili, cheese, and salt.

4. Place the halves in a baking pan and return to the oven. Select the Broil mode at 375°F temperature for 3 minutes.

5. Garnish with bacon bits, sour cream, and scallions.

**Per Serving:** Calories: 113 Cal |Protein: 9.2 g| Carbs: 13 g| Fat: 21 g

# Bacon Poppers

**Prep Time** 10 m | **Cook Time** 15 m | 4 **Servings**

- 1 strips bacon, crispy cooked

Dough:

- 2/3 cup water

- 1 tbsp. butter

- 1 tbsp. bacon fat

- 1 tsp. kosher salt

- 2/3 cup all-purpose flour

- Eggs

- oz. Cheddar cheese, shredded

- ½ cup jalapeno peppers

- A pinch pepper

- A pinch of black pepper

1.Whisk butter with water and salt in a skillet over medium heat. Stir in flour, then stir cook for about 3 minutes.

2.Transfer this flour to a bowl, then whisk in eggs and the rest of the ingredients.

3.Fold in bacon and mix well. Wrap this dough in a plastic sheet and refrigerate for 30 minutes. Make small balls out of this dough.

4.Place these bacon balls in the Air Fryer toaster oven and close the lid.

5.Select the Air Fry mode at 390°F temperature for 15 minutes. Flip the balls after 7 minutes, then resume cooking. Serve warm.

**Per Serving:** Calories: 240 Kcal| Protein: 14.9 g |Carbs: 7.1 g |Fat: 22.5 g

# Stuffed Jalapeno

**Prep Time** 10 m | **Cook Time** 10 m | 4 **Servings**

- 1 lb. ground pork sausage

- 1 (8 oz.) package cream cheese, softened

- 1 cup shredded Parmesan cheese

- 1 lb. large fresh jalapeno peppers halved lengthwise and seeded

- 1 (8 oz.) bottle Ranch dressing

1. Mix pork sausage ground with ranch dressing and cream cheese in a bowl.

2. But the jalapeno in half and remove their seeds.

3. Divide the cream cheese mixture into the jalapeno halves. Place the jalapeno pepper in a baking tray.

4. Set the Baking tray inside the Air Fryer toaster oven and close the lid.

5. Select the Bake mode at 350°F temperature for 10 minutes. Serve warm.

**Per Serving:** Calories: 168 Kcal |Protein: 9.4 g | Carbs: 12.1 g |Fat: 21.2 g

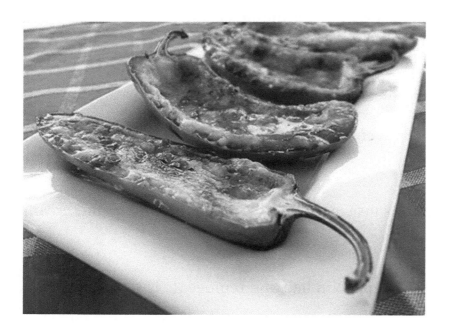

# Creamy Mushrooms

**Prep Time** 10 m | **Cook Time** 15 m | 24 **Servings**

- 20 mushrooms

- 1 orange bell pepper, diced

- 1 onion, diced

- Slices bacon, diced

- 1 cup shredded Cheddar cheese

- 1 cup sour cream

1.First, sauté the mushroom stems with onion, bacon, and bell pepper in a pan.

2.After 5 minutes of cooking, add 1 cup cheese and sour cream. Cook for 2 minutes.

3.Place the mushroom caps on the Air Fryer basket crisper plate.

4.Stuff each mushroom with the cheese-vegetable mixture and top them with cheddar cheese.

5.Insert the basket back inside and select Air Fry mode for 8 minutes at 350°F.


**Per <u>Serving:</u>** Calories: 101 Kcal |Protein: 8.8 g |Carbs: 25 g | Fat: 12.2 g

# Italian Corn Fritters

**Prep Time** 10 m | **Cook Time** 3 m | 4 **Servings**

- Cups frozen corn kernels

- 1/3 cup finely ground cornmeal

- 1/3 cup flour

- ½ tsp. salt

- ¼ tsp. pepper

- ½ tsp. baking powder

- Onion powder, to taste

- Garlic powder, to taste

- ¼ tsp. paprika

- Tbsp. green chilies with juices

- Tbsp. almond milk

- ¼ cup chopped Italian parsley

1.Beat cornmeal with flour, baking powder, parsley, seasonings in a bowl. Blend 3 tbsp. almond milk with 1 cup corn, black pepper, and salt in a food processor until smooth.

2.Stir in the flour mixture, then mixes until smooth. Spread this corn mixture in a baking tray lined with wax paper.

3.Set the baking tray inside the Air Fryer toaster oven and close the lid.

4.Select the bake mode at 350°F temperature for 2 minutes. Slice and serve.

**Per Serving:** Calories: 146 Kcal |Protein: 6.3 g| Carbs: 18.8 g| Fat: 4.5 g

# Artichoke Fries

**Prep Time** 8 m | **Cook Time** 13 m | 6 **Servings**

- 1 oz. can artichoke hearts

- 1 cup flour

- 1 cup almond milk

- ½ tsp. garlic powder

- ¾ tsp. salt

- ¼ tsp. black pepper, or to taste

For Dry Mix:

- 1 ½ cup panko breadcrumbs

- ½ tsp. paprika

- ¼ tsp. salt

1.Whisk the wet ingredients in a bowl until smooth and mix the dry ingredients in a separate bowl.

2.First, dip the artichokes quarters in the wet mixture and then coat it with the dry panko mixture.

3.Place the artichokes hearts in the Air Fryer basket. Insert the basket inside the Air Fryer toaster oven and close the lid.

4.Select the Air Fry mode at 340°F temperature for 13 minutes. Serve warm.

**Per Serving:** Calories: 199 Cal |Protein: 9.4 g |Carbs: 15.9 g |Fat: 4 g

# Crumbly Beef Meatballs

**Prep Time** 8 m | **Cook Time** 20 m | 6 **Servings**

- Lbs. of ground beef
- Large eggs
- 1-1/4 cup panko breadcrumbs
- 1/4 cup chopped fresh parsley
- 1 tsp. dried oregano
- 1/4 cup grated Parmigianino Regina
- 1 small clove garlic chopped
- Salt and pepper to taste
- 1 tsp. vegetable oil

1. Thoroughly mix beef with eggs, crumbs, parsley, and the rest of the ingredients.

2. Make small meatballs out of this mixture and place them in the basket.

3.Place the basket inside the Air Fryer toaster oven and close the lid.

4.Select the Air Fry mode at 350°F temperature for 13 minutes.

5.Toss the meatballs after 5 minutes and resume cooking.

**Per Serving:** Calories: 221 Cal |Protein: 25.1 g | Carbs: 11.2 g |Fat: 16.5 g

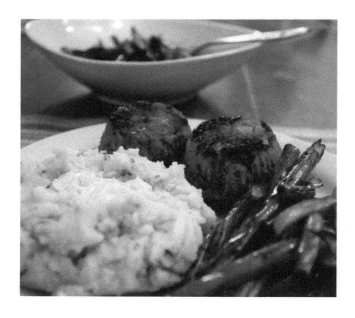

# Pork Stuffed Dumplings

**Prep Time** 15 m | **Cook Time** 12 m | 3 **Servings**

- 1 tsp. canola oil

- Cups chopped book Choy

- 1 tbsp. chopped fresh ginger

- 1 tbsp. chopped garlic

- Oz. ground pork

- 1/4 tsp. crushed red pepper

- 18 dumpling wrappers

- Cooking spray

- 1 Tbsp. rice vinegar

- 1 tsp. lower-sodium soy sauce

- 1 tsp. toasted sesame oil

- 1/2 tsp. packed light Sugar

- 1 tbsp. finely chopped scallions

1.In a greased skillet, sauté bok choy for 8 minutes, then add ginger and garlic. Cook for 1 minute.

2.Transfer the bok choy to a plate.

3.Add pork and red pepper, then mix well. Place the dumpling wraps on the working surface and divide the pork fillings on the dumpling wraps.

4.Wet the edges of the wraps and pinch them together to seal the filling.

5.Place the dumpling in the Air Fryer basket.

6.Set the Air Fryer basket inside the Air Fryer toaster oven and close the lid.

7.Select the Air Fry mode at 375°F temperature for 12 minutes.

8.Flip the dumplings after 6 minutes, then resume cooking.

**Per Serving:** Calories: 172 Cal| Protein: 2.1 g |Carbs: 18.6 g |Fat: 10.7 g

# Panko Tofu with Mayo Sauce

**Prep Time** 10 m | **Cook Time** 20 m | 4 **Servings**

- 1 tofu cutlets

- For the Marinade

- 1 tbsp. toasted sesame oil

- 1/4 cup soy sauce

- 1 tsp rice vinegar

- 1/2 tsp garlic powder

- 1 tsp. ground ginger

Make the Tofu:

- 1/2 cup vegan mayo

- 1 cup panko breadcrumbs

- 1 tsp. of sea salt

1. Whisk the marinade ingredients in a bowl and add tofu cutlets. Mix well to coat the cutlets.

93

2. Cover and marinate for 1 hour. Meanwhile, whisk crumbs with salt and mayo in a bowl.

3. Coat the cutlets with crumbs mixture. Place the tofu cutlets in the Air Fryer basket.

4. Select the Air Fry mode at 370°F temperature for 20 minutes. Flip the cutlets after 10 minutes, then resume cooking.

**Per Serving:** Calories: 151 Cal |Protein: 1.9 g | Carbs: 6.9 g |Fat: 8.6 g

# Garlicky Bok Choy

**Prep Time** 10 m | **Cook Time** 10 m | 2 **Servings**

- bunches baby book Choy

- Spray oil

- 1 tsp. garlic powder

1.Toss bok choy with garlic powder and spread them in the Air Fryer basket.

2.Spray them with cooking oil.

3.Place the basket inside the Air Fryer toaster oven and close the lid.

4.Select the Air Fry mode at 350°F temperature for 6 minutes. Serve fresh.

**Per Serving:** Calories: 81 Cal |Protein: 0.4 g | Carbs: 4.7 g |Fat: 8.3 g

# Walnut Brownies

**Prep Time** 15 m | **Cook Time** 35 m | 6 **Servings**

- Eggs 2

- Brown sugar 1 cup

- Vanilla ½ teaspoon

- Cocoa powder 1/4 cup

- Walnuts 1/2 cup, chopped

- All-purpose flour – 1/4 cup

- Butter – 1/2 cup, melted

- Pinch of salt

1.Sprinkle a baking dish with cooking spray and set aside. In a bowl, whisk together eggs, butter, cocoa powder, and vanilla. Add walnuts, flour, sugar, and salt and stir well. Pour batter into the baking dish. Place steam rack into the instant pot. Place baking dish on top of the steam rack. Seal pot with the air fryer lid. Select bake mode and cook at 320 F for 35 minutes. Serve.

**Per Serving:** Calories 340 Carbs 30g Fat 23g Protein 5g

# Seasoned Cauliflower Chunks

**Prep Time** 10 m | **Cook Time** 15 m | 4 **Servings**

- 1 cauliflower head, diced into chunks

- ½ cup unsweetened milk

- Tbsp. mayo

- ¼ cup all-purpose flour

- ¾ cup almond meal

- ¼ cup almond meal

- 1 tsp. onion powder

- 1 tsp. garlic powder

- 1 tsp. of sea salt

- ½ tsp. paprika

- Pinch of black pepper

- Cooking oil spray

1.Toss cauliflower with the rest of the ingredients in a bowl, then transfers to the Air Fryer basket.

2.Spray them with cooking oil.

3.Set the basket inside the Air Fryer toaster oven and close the lid.

4 Select the Air Fry mode at 400°F temperature for 15 minutes. 5 Toss well and serve warm.

**Per Serving:** Calories: 137 Cal |Protein: 6.1 g |Carbs: 26 g |Fat: 8 g

# Almond Butter Brownies

**Prep Time** 10 m | **Cook Time** 15 m | 4 **Servings**

- 1/2 cup Almond butter

- 1/2 teaspoon Vanilla

- 1 tablespoon Almond milk

- 2 tablespoons Coconut sugar

- 2 tablespoons Applesauce

- 2 tablespoons Honey

- 1/4 teaspoon Baking powder

- 1/2 teaspoon Baking soda

- 2 tablespoons Cocoa powder

- 3 tablespoons Almond flour

- 1 tablespoon Coconut oil

- 1/4 teaspoon Sea salt

1.Sprinkle baking pan with cooking spray and set aside. In a small bowl, mix almond flour, baking soda, baking powder, and cocoa powder and set aside. Add coconut oil and almond butter into the microwave-safe bowl and microwave until melted. Stir. Add honey, milk, coconut sugar, vanilla, and applesauce into the melted coconut oil mixture and stir well. Add flour mixture and stir to combine. Pour batter into the baking pan. Place steam rack into the instant pot. Place baking pan on top of the steam rack. Seal pot with the air fryer lid. Select bake mode and cook at 350 F for 15 minutes. Serve.

**Per Serving:** Calories 170 Carbs 22g Fat 8g Protein 2g

# Brownie Muffins

**Prep Time** 10 m | **Cook Time** 15 m | 6 **Servings**

- 1/4 cup Cocoa powder

- 1/2 cup Almond butter

- 1 cup Pumpkin puree

- 8 drops Liquid stevia

- 2 scoops of Protein powder

1.Mixed all the ingredients into the mixing bowl and beat until smooth. Pour batter into the 6 silicone muffin molds. Place the dehydrating tray into the multi-level air fryer basket and place the basket into the instant pot. Place muffin molds on a dehydrating tray. Seal pot with the air fryer lid. Select bake mode and cook at 350 F for 15 minutes. Serve.

**Per Serving:** Calories 70 Carbs 6g Fat 2g Protein 8g

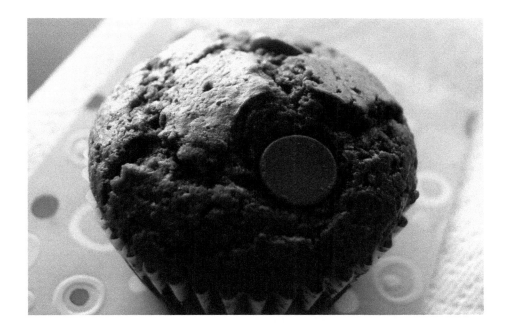

# Delicious Lemon Muffins

**Prep Time** 10 m | **Cook Time** 15 m | 6 **Servings**

- 1 Egg

- 3/4 teaspoon Baking powder

- 1 tsp. grated Lemon zest

- 1/2 cup Sugar

- 1/2 teaspoon Vanilla

- 1/2 cup Milk

- 2 tablespoons Canola oil

- 1/4 teaspoon Baking soda

- 1 cup Flour

- 1/2 teaspoon Salt

1.In a mixing bowl, beat egg, vanilla, milk, oil, and sugar until creamy. Add remaining ingredients and stir to combine. Pour batter into the 6 silicone muffin molds.

Place the dehydrating tray into the multi-level air fryer basket and place the basket into the instant pot. Place muffin molds on a dehydrating tray. Seal pot with the air fryer lid. Select bake mode and cook at 350 F for 15 minutes. Serve.

**Per Serving:** Calories 202 Carbs 34g Fat 6g Protein 4g

# Vanilla Strawberry Soufflé

**Prep Time** 10 m | **Cook Time** 15 m | 4 **Servings**

- 3 Egg whites

- 1 1/2 cup Strawberries

- 1/2 teaspoon Vanilla

- 1 tablespoon Sugar

1.Spray 4 ramekins with cooking spray and set aside. Add strawberries, sugar, and vanilla into the blender and blend until smooth. Add egg whites into the bowl and beat until medium peaks form. Add strawberry mixture and fold well. Pour egg mixture into the ramekins. Place the dehydrating tray into the multi-level air fryer basket and place the basket into the instant pot. Place ramekins on the dehydrating tray. Seal pot with the air fryer lid. Select bake mode and cook at 350 F for 15 minutes. Serve.

**Per Serving:** Calories 50 Carbs 8g Fat 0.5g Protein 3g

# Healthy Carrot Muffins

**Prep Time** 15 m | **Cook Time** 20 m | 6 **Servings**

- 1 Egg

- 1 teaspoon Vanilla

- 1/4 cup Brown sugar

- 1/4 cup Granulated sugar

- 1/2 tablespoon Canola oil

- 1/4 cup Applesauce

- 1 cup all-purpose flour

- 1 1/2 teaspoons Baking powder

- 1/2 teaspoon Nutmeg

- 1 teaspoon Cinnamon

- 3/4 cup Grated carrots

- 1/4 teaspoon Salt

1.Into a large bowl, put all the ingredients, then mix until thoroughly combined. Pour batter into 6 silicone muffin molds. Place the dehydrating tray into the multi-level air fryer basket and place the basket into the instant pot. Place muffin molds on the dehydrating tray. Seal pot with the air fryer lid. Select bake mode and cook at 350 F for 20 minutes. Serve.

**Per Serving:** Calories 165 Carbs 33g Fat 2g Protein 3g

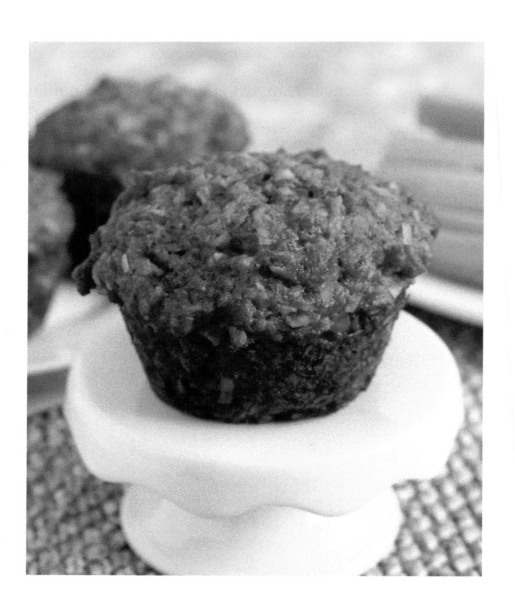

Lightning Source UK Ltd.
Milton Keynes UK
UKHW021146050321
379831UK00006B/51